I0765856

THE SIMPLE ART OF DETOXIFYING THE LIVER

A definitive liver salvage book, the ideal manage on the most proficient method to recuperate, detox and scrub your liver for a superior life

Dr. Jason Hopkins

Contents

CHAPTER ONE

What Is Liver Failure?

Liver disappointment is a perilous condition that requests critical medicinal care. Regularly, liver disappointment happens step by step, over numerous years. It's the last phase of numerous liver ailments. In any case, a rarer condition known as intense liver disappointment happens quickly (in as meager as 48 hours) and can be hard to recognize from the start.

Liver disappointment happens when enormous parts of the liver become harmed destroyed and the liver can't work any longer.

There are two sorts of live disappointment:

•   Acute: This is the point at which your liver quits working inside merely days or weeks. A great many people who get this don't have any sort liver ailment or issue before this occasion.

•   Chronic: Damage to your liver develops after some time and makes it quit working.

Manifestations of Liver Disease and Liver Failure

The early manifestations of liver disappointment are regularly like those of liver illnesses and different conditions. Along these lines, liver disappointment might be difficult to analyze from the outset. Early side effects include:

- Nausea

- Loss of craving

- Fatigue

- Diarrhea

In any case, as liver disappointment advances, the manifestations become increasingly genuine, requiring care immediately. These side effects include:

- Jaundice

- Bleeding effectively

- Swollen midsection

- Mental perplexity (known as hepatic encephalopathy)

- Sleepiness

CHAPTER TWO

Reasons For Acute Liver Failure

The reasons for intense liver disappointment, when the liver bombs quickly, include:

•	Acetaminophen overdose: Large dosages can harm your liver or lead to disappointment.

•	Viruses including hepatitis A, B, and E, the Epstein-Barr infection, cytomegalovirus, and herpes simplex infection: They lead to liver harm or cirrhosis.

•	Reactions to certain remedy and home grown drugs: Some murder cells in your liver. Others harm the pipe framework that moves bile through it.

• Eating harmful wild mushrooms: A sort called Amanita phalloides, otherwise called demise top, contains poisons that harm liver cells and lead to liver disappointment inside two or three days.

• Autoimmune hepatitis: As with viral hepatitis, this infection, where your body assaults your liver, can prompt intense liver disappointment.

• Wilson's illness: This hereditary malady keeps your

body from expelling copper. It develops in, and harms, your liver.

•   Acute greasy liver of pregnancy: In this uncommon condition, abundance fat assembles on your liver and harms it.

•   Septic stun: This mind-boggling disease in your body can harm your liver or cause it to quit working.

•   Budd Chiari disorder: This uncommon ailment limits and obstructs the bloodvessels in your liver.

• Industrial poisons: Many synthetic compounds, including carbon tetrachloride, a cleaner and degreaser, can harm your liver.

CHAPTER THREE

Reasons for Chronic Liver Failure

The most widely recognized reasons for interminable liver disappointment include:

• Hepatitis B: It makes your liver swell and prevents it from working the manner in which it should.

• Hepatitis C: If you have it long haul, it can prompt cirrhosis.

• Long-term alcoholconsumption: It likewise prompts cirrhosis.

• Hemochromatosis: This acquired issue makes your body ingest and store an excessive amount of iron. It can develop in your liver and cause cirrhosis.

Different conditions that can prompt liver disappointment include:

• Hepatitis A: Contact with nourishment or water defiled with the hepatitis An infection, or with an individual who's tainted with infection, can cause liver aggravation. This sort ordinarily leaves individually.

• Autoimmune hepatitis: In this sort, your body's invulnerable framework, not an infection, assaults your liver and causes irritation.

• Cirrhosis: Things like drinking liquor for a long time or having hepatitis scar your liver can make it hard or incomprehensible for your liver to work.

• Primary sclerosing cholangitis: This ailment gradually harms your bile channels. It for the most part influences youngsters.

• Oxalosis: This is the point at which your kidneys can't dispose of calcium oxalate precious stones through your pee.

- Wilson's ailment: People with this uncommon acquired illness store an excess of copper in their mind and liver.

- Alpha-1 antitrypsin inadequacy: This hereditary condition can prompt lung or liver malady.

- Liver malignancy: People with long haul hepatitis B or hepatitis C frequently get this.

- Liver adenoma: This is when favorable liver tumors are on a generally solid liver. This frequently influences ladies between ages 20 and 44.

• Fatty liver sickness: Extra fat cells can develop on your liver. Nonalcoholic greasy liver ailment frequently influences individuals who are overweight, stout, or have elevated cholesterol. Liquor related greasy liver malady influences overwhelming consumers.

• Alcoholic hepatitis: Liver aggravation that outcomes from substantial or long haul drinking.

• Alagille disorder: A hereditary issue that outcomes in

less bile pipes than ordinary in the liver.

• Primary biliary cholangitis (PBC): Over time, this infection obliterates your little bile channels. You may at present hear it called by its previous name, essential biliary cirrhosis.

• Galactosemia: People with this condition can't process galactose, a sugar found in numerous nourishments. It can cause liver harm.

• Lysosomal corrosive lipase lack (LAL-D): With this hereditary condition, you can't deliver a catalyst called lysosomal corrosive lipase (LAL), which enables your body to separate fats and cholesterol in your phones. Therefore, fats remain in your liver and cause harm.

CHAPTER FOUR

•   Stage 1: Inflammation. In the beginning periods, your liver will be kindled and could be delicate. Or on the other hand it may not trouble you by any stretch of the imagination.

•   Stage 2: Fibrosis/scarring. On the off chance that you don't treat the irritation, it will cause scarring. As scar tissue develops in your liver, it stops blood stream, which shields the sound parts from carrying out their responsibility and makes them work more earnestly.

- Stage 3: Cirrhosis. The scar tissue dominates, and with less and less solid tissue to carry out its responsibility, your liver won't function admirably, or it won't work by any means.

- Stage 4: End-arrange liver disappointment/illness. This is an umbrella term for a few conditions, including swollen liver, inner dying, loss of kidney work, liquid in your paunch, and lung issues. Just a liver transplant can fix it.

Tests and techniques used to analyze liver disappointment and liver malady include:

• Blood tests. These let your primary care physician know how well your liver is functioning. You may get a prothrombin time test, which estimates to what extent it takes your blood to cluster. With intense liver disappointment, blood doesn't clump as fast as it should.

• Imaging tests. These take pictures that let your primary care physician see what's happening in your liver and make sense of what's causing the issue. He may suggest

- Ultrasound

- Abdominal electronic tomography (CT) examining

- Magnetic reverberation imaging (MRI)

• Biopsy. The specialist will utilize a needle to evacuate a little bit of liver tissue and take a gander at it in the lab. A transjugular liver biopsy is an exceptional method that gives the specialist a chance to place the needle into a vein in your neck.

Medicine Acetylcysteine can turn around intense liver disappointment brought about by an acetaminophen overdose. In any case, you need to take it rapidly. There are likewise prescriptions that can switch the impacts of mushrooms or different toxins.

Steady care. On the off chance that an infection causes liver disappointment, a medical clinic can treat your side effects until the infection runs its course. In these cases, the liver will now and then recuperate without anyone else.

Liver transplant. On the off chance that your liver disappointment results from long haul harm, the initial step might be to attempt to spare whatever piece of your liver still works. On the off chance that that comes up short, you'll need a liver transplant. Luckily, this technique is frequently fruitful.

Specialists will work to anticipate inconveniences, which include:

• Cerebral edema. Liquid development is an issue with liver disappointment. Notwithstanding your gut, it can likewise pool in your mind and lead to hypertension there.

• Blood thickening issues. Your liver assumes a major job in helping your blood coagulation. At the point when it can't carry out that responsibility, you're in danger of draining too unreservedly.

• Infections, similar to pneumonia and UTIs. End-arrange liver malady can make you bound to get discases.

• Kidney disappointment. Liver disappointment can change the manner in which your kidneys work and lead to disappointment.

CHAPTER FIVE

In what manner Can Liver Failure Be Prevented?

The most ideal approach to anticipate liver disappointment is to constrain your danger of getting cirrhosis or hepatitis. Here are a few hints to help avert these conditions:

• Get a hepatitis immunization or an immunoglobulin shot to counteract hepatitis A and B.

• Eat a legitimate eating regimen from the entirety of the nutrition types.

- Maintain a sound weight.

- Do not savor liquor overabundance. Stay away from liquor when you are taking acetaminophen.

- Practice appropriate cleanliness. Since germs are generally spread by hands, make certain to wash your hands altogether after you utilize the washroom. Likewise, wash your hands before you contact any nourishment.

•	Don't share any close to home toiletry things, including toothbrushes and razors.

•	If you get a tattoo or a body puncturing, ensure the conditions are clean and all hardware is aseptic (free of malady causing germs).

•	Be sure to utilize hindrance insurance (condoms) when engaging in sexual relations.

•	If you utilize illicit intravenous medications, don't impart needles to anybody.

It's not something you most likely contemplate, however your liver is a key player in your body's stomach related framework. All that you eat or drink, including medication, goes through it. You have to treat it right so it can remain solid and carry out its responsibility.

"It's an organ you could without much of a stretch waste in the event that you don't take great consideration of it," says Rohit Satoskar, MD, of the MedStar Georgetown Transplant Institute. "What's more, when you garbage it, it's no more."

Your liver is about the size of a football and sits under your lower ribcage on the correct side. It has a few significant activities. It helps clean your blood by disposing of hurtful synthetic concoctions that your body makes. It makes fluid called bile, which causes you separate fat from nourishment. What's more, it likewise stores sugar called glucose, which gives you a speedy jolt of energy when you need it.

There's nothing dubious about keeping your liver fit as a fiddle. It's about a sound way of life, says Ray Chung, MD, restorative executive of the transplant program at Massachusetts General Hospital.

"Dealing with your liver is unquestionably more about maintaining a strategic distance from what's terrible than it is tied in with eating or drinking things that are especially feeding to the liver," he says.

Here are a few different ways to keep your liver sound:

Try not to drink a great deal of liquor. It can harm liver cells and lead to the growing or scarring that becomes cirrhosis, which can be fatal.

What amount of liquor is excessively? U.S. government rules state men should drink close to two beverages per day and ladies just one.

Eat a sound eating routine and get customary exercise. Your liver will bless your heart. You'll monitor your weight, which averts nonalcoholic greasy liver malady (NAFLD), a condition that prompts cirrhosis.

Watch out for specific drugs. Some cholesterol medications can at times have a symptom that messes liver up. The painkiller acetaminophen (Tylenol) can hurt your liver on the off chance that you take excessively.

You might be taking more acetaminophen than you understand. It's found in several medications like virus meds and remedy torment meds.

A few meds can hurt your liver on the off chance that you drink liquor when you take them. Also, some are hurtful when joined with different medications. Converse with your primary care physician or drug specialist about the most secure approach to take your prescriptions.

Figure out how to counteract viral hepatitis. It's a genuine malady that damages your liver. There are a few kinds. You get hepatitis A from eating or drinking water that is got the infection that causes the sickness. You can get an immunization in case you're heading out to a piece of the existence where there are episodes.

Hepatitis B and C are spread through blood and body liquids. To cut your hazard, don't share things like toothbrushes, razors, or needles. Farthest point the quantity of sexpartners you have, and consistently use latex condoms.

There's no immunization yet for hepatitis C, however there is one for hepatitis B.

Get tried for viral hepatitis. Since it regularly doesn't cause indications, you can have it for a considerable length of time and not know it. On the off chance that you think you've had contact with the infection, converse with your PCP to check whether you need a blood test.

Hepatitis A, B, and C spread in altogether different ways, making mellow genuine consequences for the liver.

The CDC suggests you get tried for hepatitis C in the event that you were conceived between 1945 – 1965. The person born after WW2 age is bound to have the illness.

Try not to contact or take in poisons. Some cleaning items, vaporized items, and bug sprays have synthetic concoctions that can harm your liver. Maintain a strategic distance from direct contact with them. Added substances in cigarettes can likewise harm your liver don't as well, smoke.

Be cautious with herbs and dietary enhancements. Some can hurt your liver. A not many that have caused issues are cascara, chaparral, comfrey, kava, and ephedra.

Lately, a few herbs and enhancements have hit the market that state they reestablish the liver, including milk thorn seed, borotutu bark, and chanca piedra. Be careful about those cases. "There will never be been any great proof that any of these advances liver wellbeing," Chung says. Some may even cause hurt.

Drink espresso. Research shows that it can bring down your danger of getting liver infection. Nobody knows why this is along these lines, yet it merits watching out for as more research is finished.

To keep your liver sound, pursue a solid way of life and watch out for medications, Chung says. "The liver can be an easy-going organ, yet it has its points of confinement."

One of the most widely recognized and possibly extreme symptoms of liquor addiction is liver harm, which, in serious cases, may prompt passing.

Indeed, as per the National Institute on Alcohol Abuse and Alcoholism, "A relationship between liver infection and overwhelming liquor utilization was perceived over 200 years back. Long haul overwhelming liquor use is the most common single reason for sickness and passing from liver ailment in the United States. The liver is especially helpless to liquor related damage since it is the essential site of liquor digestion."

The sooner a heavy drinker quits drinking, the happier their body will be over the long haul.

In spite of the fact that stopping liquor utilize alone won't generally fix the harm, there are different strategies one may take when endeavoring to make the liver sound once more? On the whole, it's essential to see how liquor influences the usefulness of the liver.

As indicated by Health line, the liver, which is viewed as an organ, performs numerous jobs inside the body. One of the most significant capacities is freeing the assortment of poisons and destructive substances. Moreover, the liver stores nutrients, iron, and glucose, changes over put away sugar to practical sugar when the body's sugar levels fall, separates hemoglobin and wrecks old platelets.

At the point when liquor is acquainted with the liver, it produces acetaldehyde, which is a dangerous catalyst that can harm liver cells and cause scarring. Also, liquor gets dried out the body, and the liver expects water to work accurately. At the point when the body needs water, the liver is compelled to pull in water from different sources.

As expressed by Love Your Liver, a lot of liquor can prompt an assortment of liver issues, including a greasy liver, alcoholic hepatitis, and cirrhosis of the liver.

A greasy liver happens when fat develops in the liver because of drinking beyond what the liver can deal with. Fat development can prompt aggravation and scarring, and can bring about alcoholic hepatitis.

Alcoholic hepatitis is a condition brought about by an aroused liver because of long haul liquor misuse. With this condition, the liver gets swollen and delicate. This meddles with the liver's capacity to perform basic capacities, and with time may form into a progressively genuine condition known as cirrhosis of the liver.

Cirrhosis is the name for the condition when the liver cells become so harmed that they are supplanted by scar tissue. This scar tissue influences blood stream and the progression of different liquids through the liver, meddling with its capacity to free the assortment of poisons.

CHAPTER SEVEN

Six different ways to help fix the liver

There are a few things you can do to help invert the impacts of liquor on your liver, for example,

Quit drinking.

In the event that you have been let you know have an undesirable liver, the first and most significant thing you can do is quit drinking liquor. Chopping down liquor consumption alone isn't sufficient, as even a modest quantity of liquor still requires the liver to work and may add to scarring. The best thing you can accomplish for your liver is quit drinking following discovering you have any phase of liver illness.

Make other solid way of life changes. This implies not any more smoking on the off chance that you are a smoker, and getting more fit in the event that you are overweight or stout. Alongside exorbitant liquor use, heftiness is a main source of liver infection, while cigarettes contain poisons which will add to the rotting condition of the liver. Improving these aspects of your life notwithstanding halting liquor use will give your liver a superior chance at improving its wellbeing.

A sound diet can prompt a more advantageous liver. At the point when you are not eating many handled nourishments, sugars, and immersed fat, the liver doesn't need to fill in as difficult to channel what comes through it. Furthermore, eating products of the soil prompts a more advantageous body in general.

Get your exercise in.

Aside from staying away from stoutness, practicing can help the liver in different manners. Normal exercise improves the safe framework and decreases the danger of liver malignant growth.

Indeed, even some over-the-counter drugs can be terrible for the liver when taken in overabundance. One such medicine is acetaminophen, which is frequently taken nearby prescriptions, for example, Nyquil. At the point when joined, these can get lethal, making the liver buckle down once more.

Try not to give superfluous poisons access.

The less poisons getting through your body, the better for your liver. This implies playing it safe, for example, utilizing a cover, when managing vaporized splashes, shower paints, shower bug sprays, shower fungicides, and some other type of splashed concoction. Likewise know about what synthetic substances could come into contact with your skin, and wear gloves if need be.

With regards to thinking about your body post-liquor misuse, the liver is a fundamental organ to focus on. Following these rules can improve the probability that your liver can ricochet again from the maltreatment it has persevered.

Predominance of Alcohol Use and Body Dysmorphic Disorder

Liquor can be utilized to adapt to side effects of BDD yet may exacerbate the condition. Find out about BDD and liquor misuse causes and medications.

Body dysmorphic issue (BDD) includes an outrageous and upsetting fixation on one's appearance, saw defects or blemishes. Liquor use is basic among individuals with BDD, with gauges that about 33% of individuals with BDD abuse liquor.

Despite the fact that the disposition modifying impacts of liquor can give brief alleviation from fixations and nosy musings brought about by BDD, it can keep somebody from looking for expert assistance for their condition. The co-event of liquor use and BDD is normal and ought to be viewed as when diagnosing and treating BDD.

Would alcohol be able to Use Cause Body Dysmorphic Disorder?

BDD and liquor use can be connected, however liquor is probably not going to be the sole reason for BDD.

BDD can regularly start from the get-go throughout everyday life, during youth or high school years. Much of the time, youngsters don't approach or introduction to liquor at this age. In any case, early-beginning BDD can be a hazard factor for later liquor misuse. In the event that the condition continues or starts in late puberty or early adulthood, somebody with BDD may start abusing liquor.

Creating BDD is a consequence of complex variables including character, family ancestry, and other emotional wellness conditions. Despite the fact that BDD and the utilization of liquor will in general start around a similar age, it's not likely that a solitary factor —, for example, liquor — would cause BDD. The connection among BDD and liquor relies upon character, the age the confusion started and different parts of psychological well-being.

Liquor may be utilized as an adapting procedure for BDD, yet it's not prone to cause BDD.

Does Alcohol Affect Body Dysmorphic Disorder Symptoms?

Despite the fact that it may give brief alleviation, liquor can exacerbate or draw out BDD side effects by keeping somebody from looking for expert assistance.

A portion of the sentiments and convictions related with BDD are disgrace, humiliation, and hyper-consciousness of appearance or imperfections. These indications can make it hard to work ordinarily in everyday life and especially in social circumstances. Liquor can give impermanent alleviation from these side effects, however individuals with BDD can get dependent on liquor to work.

Individuals with BDD report drinking on the grounds that having BDD is upsetting, or to assist them with foregetting about their body or appearance. Individuals with BDD can get trapped in a cycle of requiring liquor for manifestation help or to work socially. In view of this cycle, they may keep on self sedate instead of look for treatment for the basic reasons for BDD, which can delay the sickness or exacerbate it.

CHAPTER EIGHT

Can Body Dysmorphic Disorder Lead to an Unhealthy Relationship with Alcohol?

Depending on liquor for transitory alleviation from sentiments of misery and disappointment can prompt an undesirable dependence on liquor. It's been evaluated that liquor reliance in individuals with BDD may be as high as 29% and is more typical in men than ladies.

Individuals with BDD announced drinking liquor to improve how they feel about themselves and enable them to associate without consistent uneasiness about their appearance. Since liquor changes contemplations and practices, it gives transitory alleviation from fixations on appearance.

Liquor may assist somebody with BDD feel better incidentally, however it doesn't deliver basic issues identified with the confusion. Depending on liquor for manifestation help can keep somebody from looking for proficient treatment and creating sound adapting techniques.

Treatment Options for Body Dysmorphic Disorder and Co-Occurring Alcohol Addiction

The fixations, meddlesome considerations and ruminations about appearance in BDD can be troubling and can shield individuals from living their lives. Numerous individuals look for treatment for BDD through restorative or careful proceduresto change their appearance. Notwithstanding, this alternative is likely just to give impermanent help and doesn't address the fundamental issues.

Body dysmorphic issue treatment looks to address fundamental convictions about appearance and manufacture adapting abilities to oversee nosy musings and convictions. In the event that there is co-happening liquor habit, treatment should likewise address the explanations behind drinking and give new abilities and methodologies to adapt to BDD that don't include liquor.

There is a scope of treatment alternatives for BDD that can likewise address a co-happening liquor use issue. These include:

•	Medication/antidepressants, which can help decrease nosy considerations

•	Cognitive-conduct treatment, which spotlights on testing contemplations and convictions about appearance just as changing tricky practices

• Interpersonal treatment, which improves an individual's social working and connections, especially without the utilization of liquor.

THE END

www.ingramcontent.com/pod-product-compliance
Lightning Source LLC
Chambersburg PA
CBHW051415250726
48655CB00003B/1055